BIPOLAR DISORDER

A disorder associated with episodes of mood swings ranging from depression lows to maniac highs.

There is no known exact cause of bipolar disorder, but a combination of genetics, environment and altered brain structure and chemistry has a role.

Facts

- Treatment can help, but this condition can't be cured.
- Chronic: it can last for years or lifelong
- Needs medical diagnosis
- Laboratory tests or imaging not needed

Symptoms

Manic symptoms

- High energy
- Reduced need for sleep
- Loss of touch with reality

Depressive episodes

- Low energy
- Low motivation
- Loss of interest in daily activities.

Mood episodes last for days to months at a time and may also be associated with suicidal thoughts.

Treatment

Treatments are usually lifelong which in most cases combines medications and psychotherapy.

Therapy

- Support group
- Cognitive behavioral therapy
- Psychoeducation
- Family therapy

Medications

- Anticonvulsant
- Antipsychotics
- SSRIs

Palliative care

- Hospitalisation

PSYCHOSIS

A mental disorder characterized by a disconnection from reality.

Psychotic disorder may occur as a result of a psychiatric illness such as schizophrenia, health condition, medication or drug use.

Facts

- Treatable by a medical professional
- Requires a medical diagnosis
- Laboratory tests or imaging not required
- Needs emergency care

Symptoms

- Delusion
- Hallucinations
- Talking incoherently
- Agitations

Treatment

Therapy

- Cognitive behavioral therapy
- Psychoeducation
- Family therapy

Medications

- Antipsychotic

Palliative care

- Hospitalization.

SCHIZOPHRENIA

It is a disorder that affects a person's ability to think, feel and behave clearly.
There is no known precise cause of schizophrenia.

Facts

- Treatment can help, but this condition can't be cured
- Chronic: can last for years or lifelong
- Requires a medical diagnosis

Symptoms

- Disorganized speech or behavior
- Decreased participation in daily activities
- Difficulty with concentration and memory

Treatments

Treatment is usually lifelong.

Medications

- Antipsychotics
- Anti-tremor

Therapy

- Support group
- Rehabilitation

- Cognitive behavioral therapy
- Psychoeducation
- Family therapy
- Group psychotherapy

CLINICAL DEPRESSION

It is a mental health disorder characterized by persistently depressed mood or loss of interest in activities causing significant impairment in daily life.

A combination of biological, psychological and social sources of distress is a possible cause of clinical depression.

Facts

- Treatable by a medical professional
- Resolves within months
- Requires a medical diagnosis
- Lab tests or imaging are always required.

Symptoms

Changes in :
- Sleep

- Appetite
- Energy level
- Concentration
- Daily behavior
- Self-esteem

Depression can also be associated with suicidal thoughts.

Treatments

Therapy

- Cognitive behavioral therapy
- Behavioral therapy
- Psychotherapy

Medications

- SSRIs
- Antidepressants
- Anxiolytic
- Antipsychotics

Medical procedure

- Electroconvulsive therapy

ANOREXIA

An eating disorder causing people to obsess about weight and what they eat.
It is characterized by a distorted body image with an unwanted fear of being overweight.

Facts

- Treatable by a medical professional
- It can last for years or lifelong
- Usually self- diagnosable
- Lab tests or imaging not required

Symptoms

- Trying to maintain a below normal weight through starvation or too much exercise

Treatments

Therapy

- Support group
- Cognitive behavioral therapy
- Dialectical behavioral therapy
- Counseling psychology

- Interpersonal psychotherapy

Medications

- Antipsychotics
- SSRIs

VASOVAGAL SYNCOPE

A sudden drop in heart rate and blood pressure leading to fainting offer in reaction to a stressful trigger.
Common triggers include: strain, stress, long periods of standing, heat exposure, the sight of blood etc..

Facts

- Usually self-treatable
- Self-diagnosable
- Lab tests or imaging often required
- Resolves within days to weeks

Symptoms

- Paleness
- Nausea
- Sweating
- Rapid heartbeat
- Fainting.

Treatments

Palliative care

- Avoidance of triggers
- Avoidance of intravenous therapy

Therapy

- Leg muscles tensing

Device therapy

- Compression stockings

OCD(OBSESSIVE COMPULSIVE DISORDER)

Obsessive compulsive disorder is characterized by unreasonable thoughts and fears that lead to compulsive behaviors

Facts

- Treatment can help, but this condition can't be cured
- Can last for years or lifelong
- Requires a medical diagnosis
- Lab tests or imaging required

Symptoms

- Fear of germs or the need to arrange objects in a specific manner.

Treatments

Medications

- SSRIs

- Anxiolytic
- Antidepressants

Therapy

- Support group
- Cognitive behavioral therapy
- Aversion therapy
- Psychoeducation
- Rational emotive behavior therapy

BULIMIA

BULIMIA is a potentially life threatening eating disorder marked by binging, followed by methods to avoid weight gain.

Facts

- Treatable by a medical professional
- It can last for years or lifelong
- Usually self-diagnosable
- Lab tests or imaging rarely required

Symptoms

- Binder eating
- Vomiting
- Avoidance of weight gain
- Excessive exercising or fasting.

Treatments

Therapy

- Support group
- Cognitive behavioral therapy
- Counseling psychology

Medications

- SSRIs

Lifestyle

- Physical exercise.

BORDERLINE PERSONALITY DISORDER

A mental disorder characterized by unstable moods, behavior and relationship.

Facts

- Treatment can help, but the condition can't be cured
- Last for years or lifelong
- Requires a medical diagnosis
- Lab tests or imaging not required

Symptoms

- Emotional instability
- Feelings of worthlessness
- Insecurity
- Impulsivity
- Impaired social relationship

Treatments

- Cognitive behavioral therapy
- Anger management
- Dialectical behavioral therapy
- Transference focused psychotherapy

BIPOLAR II DISORDER

A type of bipolar disorder characterized by depression and hypomanic episodes
It involves at least one depressive episode lasting
At least two weeks and at least one hypomanic episode lasting at least four days.

Facts

- Treatment can help but the condition can't be cured
- Requires a medical diagnosis
- Lab tests or imaging not needed
- Can last for years or lifelong

Symptoms

- Sadness
- Hopelessness
- Irritable mood

Treatments

Therapy

- Cognitive behavioral therapy
- Psychoeducation
- Psychotherapy

Medications

- Antidepressants
- Antipsychotics
- SSRIs

ALCOHOL USE DISORDER

A chronic disease characterized by uncontrolled drinking and preoccupation with alcohol
Alcoholism is the inability to control drinking due to both a physical and emotional dependence on alcohol.

Facts

- Treatment can help but this condition can't be cured
- Usually self-diagnosable
- Lab tests or imaging not needed
- Last for years or lifelong

Symptoms

- Victim begins each day with a drink
- Feel guilty about their drinking

Treatment

- Detox

Medications

- Sedatives
- Vitamins
- Alcoholism medications

Therapy

- Support group
- Cognitive behavioral therapy
- Aversion therapy
- Family therapy.

DEMENTIA

A group of thinking and social symptoms that interfere with daily functioning.
It is not a specific disease, but a group of conditions characterized by impairment of at least two brain functions, such as memory loss and judgment.

Facts

- Treatment can help, but this condition can't be cured
- Can last for years or lifelong
- Requires a medical diagnosis
- Laboratory tests or imaging are often needed.

Symptoms

- Forgetfulness
- Limited social skills
- Impaired thinking ability

Treatment

Therapy

- Rehabilitation
- Occupational therapy

Medications

- Cognitive enhancing medications.

POST-TRAUMATIC STRESS DISORDER

A disorder characterized by failure to recover after experiencing or witnessing a terrifying event.
The condition may last for months or years with triggers that can bring back memories of the traumas accompanied by intense emotional and physical reactions.

Facts

- Treatable by a medical professional
- Resolves within months

- Requires a medical diagnosis
- Lab tests or imaging not required

Symptoms

- Nightmares
- Anxiety or depressed mood
- Heightened reactivity to stimuli

Treatments

Therapy

- Cognitive behavioral therapy
- Eye movement desensitization and reprocessing
- Exposure and response movement

Medications

- SSRIs

ANXIETY DISORDER

A mental health disorder characterized by feelings of worry, anxiety or fear that are strong enough to interfere with one's daily activities.

Examples of anxiety disorders include: panic attacks, obsessive compulsive disorder and PTSD.

Facts

- Treatable by a medical professional
- Usually self-diagnosable
- Lab tests or imaging not required

Symptoms

- Stress that is out of proportion to the impact of the event
- Inability to set aside a worry
- Restlessness

Treatments

Lifestyle drug

- Avoid alcohol
- Reduce caffeine intake
- Physical exercise
- Quitting smoking
- Relaxation technique
- Stress management
- Healthy diet.

Therapy

- Cognitive behavioral therapy
- Meditation
- Psychotherapy

Medications

- SSRIs
- Anxiolytic
- Antidepressants
- Sedatives
- Nerve pain medications.

STROKE

A stroke is a medical emergency. It is the damage to the brain from interruption of its blood supply.

Facts

- Requires a medical professional
- Laboratory tests or imaging are always required
- Treatment can help but this condition can't be cured
- Needs emergency care

Symptoms

- Trouble walking
- Difficulty in speaking and understanding
- Paralysis or numbness of the face, arm or leg

Treatment

- Alteplase
- Anticoagulant
- Statin
- Antihypertensive drug
- ACE inhibitor

Palliative care

- Cardiac monitoring

Surgery

- Carotid endarterectomy

Therapy

- Speech therapy
- Rehabilitation

- Occupational therapy
- Physical therapy

APLASIA

It is a language disorder that affects a person's ability to communicate
It can occur suddenly after a stroke or head injury or develop slowly from a growing brain tumor or disease.

Facts

- Usually self-diagnosable
- Lab tests or imaging not required
- Treatment can help, but this condition can't be cured
- Critical: needs emergency care

Symptoms

- Affects a person's ability to express and understand written and spoken language.

Treatment

- Speech therapy
- Support group
- Rehabilitation
- Group psychotherapy.